OCCASIONAL
P A P E R

Breaking the Failed-State Cycle

Marla C. Haims, David C. Gompert,

Gregory F. Treverton, Brooke K. Stearns

RAND
CORPORATION

The research described in this report was sponsored by RAND Health, the RAND National Defense Research Institute (NDRI), RAND Arroyo Center, and RAND Project AIR FORCE and was conducted within the International Security and Defense Policy Center of NDRI, a federally funded research and development center sponsored by the Office of the Secretary of Defense, the Joint Staff, the Unified Combatant Commands, the Department of the Navy, the Marine Corps, the defense agencies, and the defense Intelligence Community.

Library of Congress Cataloging-in-Publication Data is available for this publication.

ISBN 978-0-8330-4466-2

The RAND Corporation is a nonprofit research organization providing objective analysis and effective solutions that address the challenges facing the public and private sectors around the world. RAND's publications do not necessarily reflect the opinions of its research clients and sponsors.

RAND® is a registered trademark.

Published 2008 by the RAND Corporation
1776 Main Street, P.O. Box 2138, Santa Monica, CA 90407-2138
1200 South Hayes Street, Arlington, VA 22202-5050
4570 Fifth Avenue, Suite 600, Pittsburgh, PA 15213-2665
RAND URL: http://www.rand.org/
To order RAND documents or to obtain additional information, contact
Distribution Services: Telephone: (310) 451-7002;
Fax: (310) 451-6915; Email: order@rand.org

Preface

In their research and field experience, the authors have observed a wide gulf separating the treatment of the security problems of failed states from the treatment of those states' economic problems. This, in turn, may impair treatment of political problems. Such disunity of effort in assisting failed states may suboptimize resource allocation, hinder coordination, and cause important demands to be neglected. With their different backgrounds—security, economic development, political systems, health policy, and institution-building—the authors felt that, as a team, they might be able to forge an integrated, general approach to rescuing failed states, recognizing that each specific case demands a tailored approach. After holding a seminar with representatives of the World Bank, the United Nations, development agencies, and several security organizations, the RAND team set out in search of ideas that would bridge the gap and thus permit more effective strategies and actions toward failed states.

The approach on which they settled was to identify certain critical difficulties that contribute to the cycle of violence, economic collapse, and political failure that ensnares vulnerable states. While such difficulties demand special attention, they often suffer from *inattention*—precisely because they fall into the crevasses between security, economics, and politics. Simply stated, the international community is ill equipped to treat the causes of state failure.

For experts in development and security, the critical challenges flagged and solutions offered by the team may not be novel. Rather, they may reflect concerns that such experts have harbored but have been unable to tackle satisfactorily because of the jurisdictional limits, bureaucratic-cultural impediments, and disconnected funding mechanisms that form institutional gaps that experts themselves cannot bridge. Thus, while this paper should be of interest to researchers and practitioners, it is primarily intended for policymakers—legislators, senior officials in national governments, and executives in international organizations, up to and including ministers and members of governing boards—who are in a position to break down the barriers that have impeded success in breaking the failed-state cycle.

In an attempt to reach across the divide that hinders efforts to treat failed states, this work was supported by several RAND research units involved in security and development. The research was sponsored by RAND Health, the RAND National Defense Research Institute, RAND Arroyo Center, and RAND Project AIR FORCE and was conducted within the International Security and Defense Policy Center of the RAND National Defense Research Institute, a federally funded research and development center sponsored by the Office of the Secretary of Defense, the Joint Staff, the Unified Combatant Commands, the Department of the Navy, the Marine Corps, the defense agencies, and the defense Intelligence Community.

For more information on RAND's International Security and Defense Policy Center, contact the Director, James Dobbins. He can be reached by email at James_Dobbins@rand.org; by phone at 703-413-1100, extension 5134; or by mail at the RAND Corporation, 1200 South Hayes Street, Arlington, VA 22202-5050. More information about RAND is available at www.rand.org.

Contents

Figures

Tables

Summary

The Failed-State Problem

Insecurity in the 21st century appears to come less from the collisions of powerful states than from the debris of imploding ones. Failed states present a variety of dangers: religious and ethnic violence; trafficking of drugs, weapons, blood diamonds, and humans; transnational crime and piracy; uncontrolled territory, borders, and waters; terrorist breeding grounds and sanctuaries; refugee overflows; communicable diseases; environmental degradation; warlords and stateless armies. Regions with failed states are at risk of becoming failed regions, like the vast triangle from Sudan to the Congo to Sierra Leone. For security, material, and moral reasons, leading states cannot ignore failed ones.

Yet both the world's leading states and the multilateral institutions they manage are struggling in their attempts to help failed states recover. Indeed, "[t]he complex problem of state failure may be much discussed, but it remains little understood."[1] Although the sheer magnitude and multitude of the problems that failed states face go a long way toward explaining such frustration, we find (as others have) that the *linkages* among these challenges are what make recovery so difficult—linkages that the international community is not organized to treat.

What are failed states? For the purposes of this paper, they are of the sort flagged for "alert" by the Fund for Peace in its periodic Failed States Index.[2] While no two are alike, failed states typically suffer from cycles of violence, economic breakdown, and unfit governments that render them unable to relieve their people's suffering, much less empower them. Such cycles are characterized as follows:

- Violence disrupts farming, commerce, and foreign aid; diverts human resources; devours money; destroys physical infrastructure; and distracts government.
- Economic breakdown fuels conflict over resources, anger over inequality, distrust of government, factional strife, and the appeal of insurgents and extremists.
- Distrust of government damages its effectiveness and weakens popular cooperation with government programs and agents.
- Government fragility or corruption can weaken or pervert control of security forces, which may turn to marauding, death squads, or ethnic conflict.

---

[1] Fund for Peace and *Foreign Policy*, "The Failed States Index 2007," *Foreign Policy*, Vol. 161, July–August 2007, pp. 54–63.

[2] See Fund for Peace, "Failed States Index Scores 2007," Web page, 2007b, and Fund for Peace, "Failed States Index FAQ," Web page, 2007a.

- Political paralysis, arbitrariness, and exclusion undermine economic confidence, scare away investors, and destroy opportunity.
- Suffering, deprivation, inequity, and loss of livelihood breed violence among the population, strengthening the failed-state cycle.

Because of this cycle, a common feature of failed states is that the energy of their populations is consumed by the struggle for survival rather than engaged industriously in recovery. Emergency interventions—peacekeeping and humanitarian relief—may assist in survival but not durable recovery. Traditional antipoverty, development, and security-assistance programs, while helpful, are often insufficient to break the cycle that has trapped the population. Leading states (e.g., the United States and its European allies) and international organizations (e.g., the World Bank and the United Nations) are having trouble rescuing failed states not for lack of concern, which is growing, but because their efforts are too fragmented.

Integrating Strategy

This paper aims to improve the understanding and treatment of failed states by offering an integrated approach based on two ideas:

- First, certain *critical challenges* at the intersections between security, economics, and politics must be met if the cycle is to be broken.
- Second, in meeting these critical challenges, the guiding goal should be to *lift the population* from the status of victims of failure to agents of recovery.

Our work has revealed that both ideas imply a higher degree of integration in recovery efforts than the international community is currently capable of providing.

Identifying critical challenges is key. Generally speaking, breaking the cycle and enabling the populations of failed states requires (1) dismantling instruments of violence, (2) removing incentives for violence, and (3) creating security for economic recovery. Under these broad headings, six critical challenges and ways of meeting them can be identified.

Critical Challenges

While the exact challenges of a failed state are determined by specific circumstances, those that follow are typical. They will be familiar to most practitioners and scholars who deal with failed states. Our point is not that these challenges are unknown but that they are not given the actual effort that their criticality warrants.

Dismantling Instruments of Violence

1. Educating, training, and rehabilitating excombatants (on all sides) for civilian life or duty in reformed security services:
   - Excombatants are a large pool of people who can either perpetuate violence or become agents of recovery, depending on whether they are integrated.

- Literacy and other basic schooling are vital first steps for both adult and child excombatants. Beyond this, job training and placement services are needed.
- Legal, social, and political rehabilitation—except when serious crimes have been committed—can offer a more promising future than can retribution.

2. Reforming "power" agencies that oversee national security services:
   - Dissolving and rebuilding security forces, though costly, has been routinely accomplished throughout history. But if the agencies that control security—departments and ministries of defense, interior, justice, and intelligence—are not also reformed, state power will remain subject to abuse, and political reform will remain fragile.
   - Security-sector reform must give as much attention to these institutions as it does to organizing, training, and equipping military and police forces.
   - Building efficient, fair, and transparent justice systems is indispensable to legitimacy, law, and order—and thus to security itself. Yet this is one of the most glaring deficiencies in both international capability and execution.

Removing Incentives for Violence

3. Distributing aid widely and appropriately to create shared equity in recovery:
   - Failed states are usually divided societies. When violence stops but cleavages remain, the chances are high that the state will reenter a cycle of failure.
   - Both emergency and development aid should be distributed fairly, widely, and where people live. It should include efforts to encourage production and to build local and provincial institutions that foster public trust in government.
   - Development planning should offer opportunities for local initiative. Depending on the fault lines of the population, planning can help heal differences via functional and economic domains in which common interests can be addressed.

4. Instituting inclusive and representative politics:
   - Victims of the "politics of exclusion" often seek influence or redress through violence and insurgency. To be and to be perceived as legitimate, a government needs multiparty elections, anticorruption efforts, civil-service reform, and accountability.
   - Provincial and local politics are vital to enhancing inclusion, responsiveness, and empowerment, giving the entire population some stake in recovery.
   - Such involvement should feed into national-development planning.

Creating Security for Economic Recovery

5. Securing critical economic resources and infrastructure:
   - The security of key natural resources, transport routes, ports and airstrips, power grids, pipelines, industry hubs, and marketplaces must be a high priority for local and foreign security forces. These are favored targets for insurgents, extremists, warlords, crime lords, and other spoilers.
   - At the same time, sufficient funds must be invested in the security sector: An absence of financial and material resources can lead to bribery, dissent, and abuse by the very individuals meant to uphold law, order, and security.

- These measures, including the development of a visible and professional police force, can reduce violence against and conflict over economic assets, offer jobs, strengthen state authority and revenues, and create physical conditions in which human resources can thrive.

6. Offering safe conditions for early foreign direct investment:
   - Failed-state conditions—violence, economic collapse, and political stalemate or turmoil—are anathema to foreign investors. Besides creating physical safety, the recovering state and its external supporters should move promptly to create conditions hospitable to foreign investment through investment incentives, contract and property law, security from appropriation, and support for trade.
   - Potential investors will expect not only security but also government effectiveness and integrity. Because they will be seeking advantages in global markets, the ability to get materials in and goods out must be assured, which requires protection from threats and interference.

Because these critical challenges bear on the cycle of violence, economic breakdown, and unfit government, they must be tackled aggressively and more or less concurrently. Yet, because they do not fit within traditional security, development, and governance domains, they may be neglected in failed-state recovery efforts. For example, reintegrating excombatants requires security agencies to disarm and demobilize them and economic agencies to prepare them for nonviolent livelihoods—a handoff that has failed again and again. Optimizing defense capabilities and measures to safeguard critical economic resources, markets, and investments demands closer integration of security and development strategies than is currently possible.

Generally speaking, the reason such prescriptions often fall through the cracks is less the result of a lack of awareness on the part of security and development practitioners than of institutional and funding barriers and gaps that limit integrated action. Meeting these critical challenges will thus require unprecedented cooperation among security, development, and political institutions—national and multilateral—and determination among the leading states that run these institutions.

Fostering Human Industry

Meeting such critical challenges is necessary but not sufficient for rescuing failed states. For lasting recovery to occur, the industry of the local population is crucial. However, populations in danger and misery cannot transform themselves into agents of recovery. Therefore, hand in hand with actions to break the failed-state cycle by concentrating on critical challenges, recovery requires concerted efforts to replenish human confidence, energy, and productivity. As a first step, the basic needs of the population (e.g., shelter, potable water, sanitation, health care) must be met. Second, plans for sustainable human-centric development must be devised and implemented (e.g., rehabilitating secondary education, implementing usable-skill training, creating safe and accessible workplaces and marketplaces, creating security for foreign trade).

Meeting the population's basic needs and ensuring long-term development both depend on a capable and reliable central government, which failed states typically lack. Thus, it is incumbent upon international donors and other external actors to build capacity, accountability, efficiency, effectiveness, and trust within the country's government as part of all recovery initiatives.

Conclusion

Failed states can recover. Policies and resources aimed at meeting critical challenges, such as the six offered in this paper, can break the cycles of violence, economic collapse, and unfit government. As these cycles are broken, populations can rise from victims of failure to agents of recovery. For this to happen, though, institutional and resultant strategy gaps must be closed. Failed states do not conform to the way in which the international community is organized: They do not respect the boundary between security and development. Until the international community can address more squarely the reasons that states fail and cannot recover, the problem will persist and could worsen.

Our belief that the failed-state problem, in general, can be reduced is contingent on the political will and wisdom of the world's leading states—the Atlantic and East Asian democracies and the rising economic powers—to align their multilateral and national institutions to improve their approach to the problem. Although these leading states are increasingly aware of the dangers posed by failed states, other threats may seem more urgent. It will take the determination of political leaders, motivated by a sense of global order and human responsibility, to raise and keep the problem higher on their agendas and to insist on better institutional alignment and collaboration. We hope that, by illustrating effective strategies, this paper will foster such determination.

Acknowledgments

This work was prompted by a scenario-based fragile-states exercise that RAND conducted for the World Bank. We commend the Fragile States and Conflict-Affected Countries Group at the World Bank for its insights into the need for such an exercise and its desire to bridge the security-development divide that is so debilitating in the failed-state context. We are especially thankful to Laura Bailey, senior operations specialist, who worked in close partnership with RAND on the exercise.

We are grateful for the generous support provided by several RAND research units and centers that allowed us to develop and publish this paper. Funding support was provided by RAND Health, the RAND National Defense Research Institute, RAND Arroyo Center, and RAND Project AIR FORCE.

Finally, we are particularly appreciative of Sarah Cliffe of the World Bank and our RAND colleagues C. Richard Neu and James Dobbins for their valuable insights and feedback on an earlier draft of this document. Their constructive comments certainly led to an improved product. We would also like to thank Barbara Meade for her editing assistance.

Any errors are the responsibility of the authors and not of any who assisted our efforts.

Abbreviations

CDC	Centers for Disease Control and Prevention
DFID	UK Department for International Development
DRC	Democratic Republic of the Congo
G8	Group of Eight
IMF	International Monetary Fund
ODA	official development assistance
OECD	Organization for Econonomic Co-Operation and Development
PPP	purchasing-power parity
USAID	U.S. for International Development

CHAPTER ONE

Introduction

Understanding Failed States

Sudan. Iraq. Afghanistan. Somalia. Gaza. Colombia. Lebanon. Democratic Republic of the Congo (DRC). Insecurity in the 21st century derives less from the collisions of powerful states than from the debris of imploding ones. Failed states present a variety of dangers: religious and ethnic violence; trafficking in drugs, weapons, blood diamonds, and humans; transnational crime and piracy; uncontrolled territory, borders, and waters; terrorist breeding grounds and sanctuaries; refugee overflows; communicable diseases; environmental degradation; warlords and stateless armies.[1] Regions with failed states are at risk of becoming failed regions, like the vast African triangle from Sudan to the Congo to Sierra Leone. Alarmingly, two nuclear states, Pakistan and North Korea, are deemed to be among the most vulnerable states.[2] The number of failed states is long and growing; the stakes are high and rising.

For our purposes, failed states are of the sort identified by the Fund for Peace in its Failed States Index,[3] which is based on 12 indicators of state vulnerability: (1) mounting demographic pressures, (2) massive movement of refugees or internally displaced persons creating complex humanitarian emergencies, (3) legacy of vengeance-seeking group grievance or group paranoia, (4) chronic and sustained human flight, (5) uneven economic development along group lines, (6) sharp and/or severe economic decline, (7) criminalization and/or delegitimization of the state, (8) progressive deterioration of public services, (9) suspension or arbitrary application of the rule of law and widespread violation of human rights, (10) security apparatus operating as a "state within a state," (11) rise of factionalized elites, and (12) intervention of other states or external political actors.[4] In 2007, there were 32 countries in the "alert" zone based on this index.[5] These countries have experienced the greatest erosion of state capacity and economic prospects and the highest presence of or propensity for violent conflict. The majority of them also meet the World Bank's criteria for "fragile states." The World Bank uses the phrase *fragile states* to describe states characterized by economic and social deterioration, prolonged

---

[1] Paul Collier, V. L. Elliott, Håvard Hegre, Anke Hoeffler, Marta Reynal-Querol, and Nicholas Sambanis, *Breaking the Conflict Trap: Civil War and Development Policy*, Washington, D.C.: World Bank and Oxford University Press, 2003.

[2] Fund for Peace and *Foreign Policy* (2007).

[3] See Fund for Peace (2007b).

[4] Each indicator has a 10-point scale with 1 being the lowest intensity (most stable) and 10 being the highest intensity (least stable). Countries with an aggregate score above 90 are in the "alert" zone; countries with an aggregate score between 60 and 89.9 are in the "warning" zone; those with an aggregate score between 30 and 59.9 are in the "monitoring" zone; those with aggregate scores of 29.9 or below are in the "sustainable" zone.

[5] Fund for Peace (2007a). See the appendix for a list of these states and additional details.

political impasse or crisis, postconflict burdens, and little scope for rapid improvement or development.

Understanding failed states requires understanding the web of violence, economic breakdown, and unfit government that ensnares them.

- *Security:* Failed states may be descending into, in the midst of, or just coming out of conflict—usually internal but occasionally external or both. This may be characterized by lawlessness, in the form either of a breakdown of order or of order maintained, at great cost, by an unlawful government. Such lawlessness may cause or result from "organized" bloodshed, such as insurgency, deadly politics, group-on-group violence, state-sponsored militias, brutal state security services, and cross-border conflict. Usually, the severity of violence combined with the incompetence or complicity of government means that some form of international military intervention is required to establish and keep peace. The presence of U.S. forces in Iraq, NATO forces in Afghanistan, and UN forces in the DRC imply that those states are incapable of providing for their internal security, with deleterious effects on economics and politics.
- *Economy:* Failed states do not meet the preconditions of standard models of economic development. Curing poverty is difficult even in peaceful states. However, the economic consequences of violence—farming disrupted, crops destroyed, workers turned into fighters, transportation routes and marketplaces attacked, populations uprooted, supply chains disturbed, foreign visitors threatened—make failed states difficult to assist. Some failed states are moving backward economically, as evidenced by the destruction of forested and arable land, infrastructure deterioration, and rising chronic unemployment. Even when failed states are not impoverished, their ability to utilize resources to make economic progress is severely retarded. For example, Sudan and Iraq (with rankings of 1 and 2, respectively, on the 2007 Failed States Index)[6] have profited greatly from high oil prices, yet both are clearly failing.
- *Government:* As both a cause and consequence of insecurity and economic failure, the government systems of failed states cannot reliably provide services, safety, or basic administrative functions. People living in failed states usually lack the empowerment to drive necessary reforms or regime changes. Moreover, because the governments of many failed states are authoritarian, corrupt, and ineffective, they present a serious obstacle to external assistance efforts. They may waste or divert aid, as have the Fatah-led Palestinian administration and Idriss Déby's administration in Chad, or act in ways that make themselves ineligible for aid, as have Robert Mugabe's in Zimbabwe and Kim Jong Il's in North Korea.

Policy Failures

The critical importance of the failed-state problem is now widely recognized. Lately, several factors have deepened worries about failed states in policy and political circles. Anxiety about the spread of violent Islamic extremism and the staging of terrorist attacks from ungoverned areas of such states has entered U.S. strategic thinking. So has new awareness that some regions

---

[6] Fund for Peace (2007b).

containing failed states, such as West Africa and Central Asia, also contain valuable natural resources, including oil and gas. Transcending these specific security and material interests, the contrast between the advancement of much of humankind over the past two decades of globalization and the fact that citizens of failed and vulnerable states are instead moving backward does not provide for an acceptable global future—and may not be a sustainable one either.

A consensus has emerged that the world cannot write off failed states like a company shedding its unproductive assets. Somalia was essentially divested by the international community after the ill-fated UN-U.S. attempt to save it in the early 1990s, and today it is back on the agenda, with radical Islamist insurgents, Ethiopian armed intervention, and heightened dangers for the rest of Horn of Africa. Failed states do not disappear: They keep failing, often worsen over time, and sometimes infect their regions.

On the other hand, generous financial aid, in most cases, has not transformed failed states into successful ones. As evidence mounts that failed states can have serious consequences, leading powers (e.g., the United States, the European Union) and international organizations (e.g., the United Nations, the World Bank) have increased their support. According to Organization for Economic Co-Operation and Development (OECD) data, the average official development assistance (ODA) extended in 2006 to the 32 countries in the alert zone was $1,371 million, while the same states received an average of $278 million in ODA in 2000.[7] Yet, even when a large amount of aid is furnished, as it has been in Iraq and Lebanon, the results are often disappointing.

Failed states do not conform to the Western conception of effective sovereign states, and so they are perplexing to the states that provide assistance. The 2007 Failed States Index addresses this issue: "The complex problem of state failure may be much discussed, but it remains little understood."[8] Just as security strategists have had no good answers to the violence in failed states, international-development experts have been stumped by the resistance of such states to traditional development methods.

Developing an Integrated Approach

Given that failed states suffer from a cycle of violence, economic breakdown, and unfit government, helping them achieve lasting recovery requires an *integrated* program of security, economic reconstruction, and government reform. On this there is general agreement. In practice, however, integrating policies, actions, and resource decisions across the divide between security and development is difficult for any government. Doing so is both more critical and harder in failed states, where competition for resources is fierce, institutions are frail, and politics can be deadly.

What is decisive in saving failed states is not the scale of aid but how it is applied and the policies it supports. Funds are often wasted when appropriate policies are not in place. Policies tend to be narrowly devised to treat specific security or economic problems without sufficient regard for the connections between them that drive the failed-state cycle. International responsibilities and capabilities for helping failed states exist in two parallel universes: security and

---

[7]   Average ODA reported here is based on ODA to all 32 countries except North Korea, for which data are not available. See the appendix for a list of these states and their respective ODA amounts.

[8]   Fund for Peace and *Foreign Policy* (2007).

development. Bifurcated, the international community is not organized to meet the common, central challenge of breaking the cycle.

The structural problem reflects an analytic one. Security and development institutions are aware of the need to improve coordination, collectively set recovery strategies and resource priorities, and sequence measures for maximum effect. But they are largely ignorant, or naïve, about each other's domain, and they have no unified failed-state strategy framework to inform policy, coordination, and resource allocation.

Recognizing that every failed state calls for different, tailored treatment, this paper suggests a framework that integrates policies designed to strengthen security, reconstruct the economy, and rebuild the government. To this end, it

- reframes the traditional sector-by-sector approach to one more conducive to integration by diagnosing the cycle of insecurity, economic collapse, and unfit government and by placing the population at the center of this cycle
- disaggregates the failed-state cycle into specific critical challenges to recovery
- prescribes responses to these critical challenges
- identifies conditions and strategies for lasting recovery.

Throughout, the population—its condition, potential, and enhancement—is our point of reference for planning and gauging progress toward recovery. The approach focuses on strategies that enable "human industry"—the people's ability to sustain productive work to create goods, services, better lives, civil communities, and, thus, viable states. The people of failed states should not be viewed only as victims whose suffering must be relieved, but also as vital resources whose potential can be unlocked by creating the right conditions. Compared to the industry of humans, other resources—oil, land, gems, minerals, timber, rubber, and so on—are secondary.[9] Perhaps this focus on human industry is obvious—for instance, Amartya Sen argues for a freedom-centered, agent-oriented view of development[10]—but discipline in making it the standard of success has not been evident in international efforts to rescue failed states.

For a failed state's people to become agents of recovery, minimum conditions for survival first have to be met, such as by peacekeeping or humanitarian relief—usually both. Accordingly, this paper presupposes and therefore does not address emergency measures aimed at the bare survival of failed-state populations. Its premise is that the people themselves can become an increasingly important resource for recovery as their basic needs are met, conditions improve, and enabling environments are established, transforming victims of failure into agents of recovery.

---

[9]   The best evidence of this is the unimpressive record of states that are well endowed with natural resources but neglect their human resources, such as the DRC, and, conversely, the success of states endowed with productive populations but few natural resources, such as Singapore.

[10]   Amartya Sen, *Development as Freedom*, New York: Anchor Books, 1999.

CHAPTER TWO

Reframing the Failed-State Challenge

Failed states are often plagued by a combination of corruption, predatory elites, tribal feuding, ethnic persecution, religious intolerance, strongman (but otherwise weak) government, extreme poverty, or the absence of the rule of law. These problems reinforce each other and can deepen over time. Figure 2.1 depicts the vicious failed-state cycle of violence, economic collapse, and unfit government.

Traditional approaches to the failed-state challenge are usually conceived in sectors. Key sectors of response activity, along with the typical challenges faced within each, are outlined in Table 2.1.

While sector-based analysis is useful in understanding conditions, sector-limited policies are not adequate to disrupt the cycle of violence, economic breakdown, and unfit government that is the defining characteristic of failed states. Although aid organizations, such as the World Bank, regional banks, the UK Department for International Development (DFID), and the U.S. Agency for International Development (USAID), have long recognized the need

Figure 2.1
The Cycle Characterizing Failed States

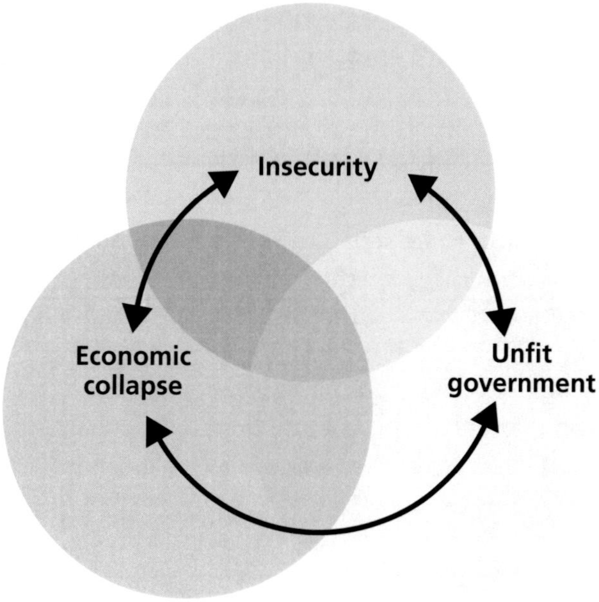

RAND *OP204-2.1*

Table 2.1
Key Sectors and Related Challenges of Traditional Recovery Efforts

Sector	Challenges
Security	Lack of law enforcement and public safety Organized, armed internal groups External and cross-border threats Land mines and other perils
Public infrastructure	Dilapidated transport infrastructure Inadequate energy and power Lack of safe drinking water and sanitation systems
Economic development	Lack of investment Collapsed agriculture, infrastructure, and markets Unemployment Inequitable distribution of opportunity and wealth
Health	Malnutrition Spreading of disease Lack of access to drugs and health care
Education	Illiteracy Lack of access to primary and secondary education
Justice	Inconsistent rule of law Lack of appropriate correctional facilities Need for truth and reconciliation
Government	Corruption and lack of accountability Lack of depoliticization and professionalism Imbalanced distribution of power
Politics	Weakened democratic processes and civil society Unruly political parties

for an integrated strategy across development sectors, the larger and thornier problem—only more recently being recognized—is that of integration across security, development, and government reform.[1] Field coordination among involved countries and agencies, while essential, is no substitute for strategic integration; conversely, it takes integrated strategy to make coordination truly productive.

Figure 2.2 depicts the concept of breaking the failed-state cycle by targeting the critical challenges that lie at the intersections of the cycle—represented in the overlap of insecurity, economic collapse, and unfit government.

This approach also requires some standard by which to qualify responses, set priorities, and measure outcomes. None of the individual sector goals—minimizing violence, maximizing GDP growth, achieving effective and legitimate government—alone is adequate. Rather, we suggest that the most appropriate standard is *industry* (as broadly defined earlier) of the local population. Choosing this standard recognizes that genuine and lasting recovery must be both measured by the condition of the people and powered by their productivity.

---

[1]   For example, the World Bank is developing a training exercise aimed at overcoming compartmentalization. The UK government is trying to address segmentation through its global fund, which is managed by DFID, the Ministry of Defence, and the Foreign and Commonwealth Office.

Figure 2.2
Breaking the Failed-State Cycle by Targeting Critical
Challenges

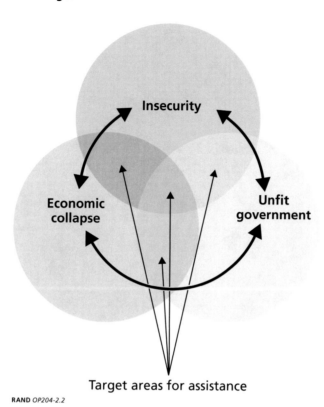

RAND *OP204-2.2*

The human conditions that result from the failed-state cycle can be generalized as

- *exposure to danger and suffering:* gang and insurgent attacks, rampant disease, and acute deprivation of nutrition, clean water, sanitation, and other daily needs of individuals, families, and communities
- *lack of opportunity:* little chance for livelihood creation, compounded by lost confidence in the state and in the future
- *unresponsive government:* absence of a functional and trustworthy state authority and administration able to address the population's suffering and hopelessness and thus earn its cooperation.

Therefore, policies and resources should be directed, above all, at reversing these conditions.

In sum, enabling states to emerge from failure requires integrated strategies to break the failed-state cycle and bolster the well-being and industry of the population. Such strategies cannot be formed or executed by institutions working apart.

CHAPTER THREE

Identifying and Meeting Critical Challenges

How can the goals described in the previous chapter be translated into practical policies and investments?

Identifying critical challenges is key. Three conditions for breaking the cycle and enabling the people of failed states are dismantling instruments of violence, removing incentives for violence, and creating security for economic recovery. Within these, we have identified six critical challenges that, if unmet, will leave the failed-state cycle unbroken. The critical challenges tend not to fall neatly into one or another traditional sector and often cross the boundaries between security, development, and government reform, which helps explain why the international community has not been especially successful at diagnosing or treating them. While the list of failed-state challenges is not exhaustive, it is indicative of what it takes to break the cycle.

In addition, this chapter includes suggested responses to each challenge, providing insights on how to better organize and employ international capabilities to help failed states emerge from failure. Needless to say, actual strategies must be tailored to the circumstances of any given failed state. The general responses suggested here are guided, above all, by the centrality of populations in recovery. They have been developed with several criteria in mind: *contribution* to general and lasting recovery, *effectiveness* under the aggravated conditions encountered in failed states, and *urgency*, given that conditions may worsen if unattended. In the analysis leading to this paper, we dropped possible responses that do not meet these criteria, sharing only those that do.

Dismantling the Instruments of Violence

Critical Challenge 1: Reintegrating Excombatants
Excombatants who remain rootless almost guarantee a fresh cycle of violence, and failed states often have excombatants in large numbers—renegade state forces, militias, insurgent forces, or armed gangs. In Liberia, for example, the estimated number of excombatants is 100,000 in a country of around 3 million people. In Iraq, the number is on the order of 600,000 in a country of 25 million. When they no longer have each other to fight, excombatants may turn to preying on the population. Depending on how long the country has been in conflict, excombatants may have little experience other than fighting, leaving them uneducated, unskilled, and unprepared for alternative lives. Worse, many failed states, especially in Africa, have large numbers of child excombatants. While they may or may not be good fighters, they are all too often seasoned killers. Rootless excombatants are a ready source of manpower (or boypower) for demagogues seeking their own goals.

In theory, programs to *disarm* and *demobilize* excombatants are meant to set the stage for *reintegration* (so-called disarmament, demobilization, and reintegration). In practice, although disarming and demobilizing may proceed more or less smoothly, timely reintegration usually proves elusive. In Liberia, for example, excombatants turned in large numbers of weapons; however, there were not sufficient resources left over for a full-scale reintegration program,[1] resulting in a latent threat to Liberia's security. Similarly, in Iraq, agreements to dissolve party-based militias failed for a lack of reintegration programs.

Response: Education, Job Training, and Employment. Of all the measures that may be taken to reintegrate excombatants, education and training are paramount. In the human-centered framework suggested here, turning large numbers of individuals from instruments of destruction into participants in recovery can have a pivotal effect. But *each individual* must be given the ability to make that shift.

A worthy objective for failed states is to provide as many excombatants as possible, regardless of the side on which they fought, with basic education and skills to pursue new work and a new life. At a minimum, this means offering literacy training to both adults and children. Illiteracy is a huge problem for many excombatants because they have fought during the years in which they should have been in school. This suggests that education programs—opening lower schools throughout the country—should be made readily accessible to excombatant children. It also suggests a need for adult literacy education, a commendable measure in any case. A meaningful target for recovery should be to raise literacy rates among excombatants to the national average as quickly as possible. In addition, job training relevant to the national or local economy can offer an alternative path that many combatants never had. While there is no guarantee that being in school will keep excombatants from crime and violence, getting them "off the street" can only help.

An equally critical issue is employment. Should jobs be created specifically for excombatants, particularly upon completion of education or training programs? Unless employed in more rewarding activities, excombatants, trained or not, may fall prey to the cycle of violence. On the other hand, giving preference to excombatants is arguably unfair to job-seekers who did not fight and may even have been victims of violence. Generally speaking, creating skills and conditions conducive to economic growth is preferable to job creation. But certain lesser measures could be helpful:

- *Job-placement services*, short of guaranteed employment, are a good way to attract excombatants while leaving to each individual the responsibility for finding work.
- *Economic state-owned enterprises* that can employ excombatants should not be dismantled until general economic conditions improve significantly.
- *Public investment and foreign aid* could be concentrated in areas where otherwise high excombatant unemployment is certain.

Response: Recruiting Excombatants for Reformed State Security Services. New state security services are critical for any failed state; the old ones are likely to have been corrupt, ineffective, politicized, or brutal. But should the new services recruit former combatants from all sides? Can those who were part of the problem be part of the solution? Cooperating with

---

[1]   David C. Gompert, Olga Oliker, Brooke K. Stearns, Keith Crane, and K. Jack Riley, *Making Liberia Safe: Transformation of the National Security Sector*, Santa Monica, Calif.: RAND Corporation, MG-529-OSD, 2007.

the local population calls upon very different skills and methods than does brutalizing fellow citizens.

The decision is not easy. If excombatants are to be recruited for reformed state security services, large and intensive reorienting and retooling programs are required. Such an investment must be weighed against the costs and uncertainties of starting over with untarnished but also inexperienced recruits. Moreover, excluding excombatants leaves them free to join new gangs or insurgencies. Shifting fighters from creating insecurity to creating security could be instrumental in breaking the failed-state cycle.

If former combatants are brought into new security forces, breaking down excombatant command chains and loyalties is crucial, making individual recruitment, as opposed to unit recruitment, imperative. Integrating individuals from diverse armed groups, factions, and forces into unified state security services is likely to be resisted, but it is essential. Moreover, new security services should not be monopolized by members of the former ones; therefore, recruitment of non-excombatants is also important.

Response: Political, Social, and Legal Rehabilitation. Which combatants should be rehabilitated? In failed states, it can be particularly difficult to distinguish deserving from undeserving excombatants. In Côte d'Ivoire, the DRC, and Sudan, for example, one is hard pressed to decide whether government forces and government-allied militias are better or worse than the several rebel forces fighting them. In Sierra Leone, Revolutionary United Front rebels chopped off the limbs of innocents. In Afghanistan and Iraq, prior to the U.S. invasions, government forces (of the Taliban and Ba'athist governments, respectively) caused most of the carnage. In Liberia, all forces committed atrocities. Punishing "losers" and rewarding "winners" is fraught with risk and potential injustice.

As a general rule, it is probably best to treat all excombatants similarly, except in cases in which serious prosecutable crimes have been committed. Accordingly, amnesty, nondiscrimination, and rehabilitation are important measures in breaking the vicious failed-state cycle and keeping it broken. These political and legal steps require strong and enlightened leadership, such as that of Liberia's Ellen Johnson-Sirleaf. They also entail some compromise of accountability and justice, which are no trifling matters. Still, on balance, excluding and stigmatizing large numbers of excombatants is a recipe for trouble: Witness the major role of Sunni former members of Saddam's security services in the current insurgency in Iraq.

Creating pathways for all excombatants to participate responsibly in the new political order can help contribute to the human capital available for recovery. Announcing amnesty and nondiscrimination in training or employment as soon as possible after a cease-fire or political agreement can serve as an inducement for excombatants to choose a future different from their past.

Critical Challenge 2: Building Effective, Legitimate State Security Structures

Reintegrating excombatants is part of an even greater challenge: building new security structures. Often, the failed state's own misuse of security organizations is an integral part of the failed-state cycle. For instance, prior RAND work on Iraq and Liberia made clear that the old security institutions and forces there were ineffective, politicized, corrupt, and unprofessional from top to bottom and across all agencies.[2] These power institutions are both prizes and tools

---

[2] Gompert et al. (2007); Olga Oliker, Keith Crane, Audra K. Grant, Terrence K. Kelly, Andrew Rathmell, and David Brannan, *U.S. Policy Options for Iraq: A Reassessment*, Santa Monica, Calif.: RAND Corporation, MG-613-AF, 2007.

of politics in dysfunctional states. The entity that controls the interior ministry and the police can be the final arbiter of politics—unless, of course, the defense ministry controls an army with yet more muscle. The head of the intelligence service or, often, multiple and competing intelligence services, typically has dossiers that can be used perniciously. New governments cannot win the trust of the people when the organizations that hold the state's "hard power" are malevolent, incompetent, or both.

The challenge of building new institutions is compounded by the scarcity of professional skills and ethics. In most failed states, only "the colonels" know how to use forces, whether responsibly or not. Failed or despotic states also often harbor symbiotic pairings of politicians who seek to use armed power for their advantage and military officers who enable them to do so in exchange for a political or economic price.

Responses: Dissolving or Reforming Failed-State Security Forces. There has been sharp debate about the U.S. decision to abolish the Iraqi army following the 2003 invasion. Defenders of the decision point out that the army was a powerful instrument and indelible symbol of Saddam's reign of terror against his own people, especially the Shi'ite Arabs and Kurds, who comprise four-fifths of the population. Critics claim that what postinvasion Iraq needed most was hundreds of thousands of Iraqi soldiers to blanket the country and guard its borders under U.S. control, and what it needed least was hundreds of thousands of dismissed, stigmatized, alienated veterans, especially the Sunni-dominated officer corps, free to turn to insurgency.

A parallel U.S. decision has been less discussed. The United States retained Iraq's police force, despite its well-deserved reputation among the people for incompetence and corruption. The hope that abbreviated retraining of a large, unprofessional police force would produce a professional one proved to be an illusion; five years later, Iraq's police force is plagued by ineffectiveness and worse—sectarian death squads. (The new army, in contrast, is *comparatively* professional and nonsectarian.)

This tale of two forces—the Iraqi police and the Iraqi military—illustrates a serious dilemma in failed-state recovery strategy: whether to overhaul or instead dissolve and build anew the indigenous forces on which the state depends for security. One or the other is imperative, but it is impossible to decide in the abstract which option is better. It depends on

- whether the officer corps as a whole has been compromised
- how much trust and confidence the population has in the forces
- whether atrocities have been committed
- the extent of training needed under each option
- the time, cost, and likelihood of success of each option.

All else being equal, replacing old armies with new ones is not as problematic as replacing old police forces with new ones. Depending on security conditions, including the presence of peacekeepers, a country may be able to make do without an army while a new one is being built. Police, in contrast, have an essential role in everyday public order and safety; therefore, removing even inferior ones can cause crime and violence to rise—hardly helpful when trying to help a failed state recover.[3] Moreover, armies have (or should have) narrower roles than do police, as well as clearer international standards to facilitate building them anew. Experience

---

[3]   Recognizing this, the UN is placing greater emphasis on international police forces to replace or augment local police.

in Afghanistan conforms to experience in Iraq: It is harder for outsiders to build a new police force than a new army.

In any case, the choice to disband or reform is too important to be driven by short-term expediency (e.g., with decisions based on personalities or factionalism). Getting it wrong can have devastating consequences. To promote good decisions and plans for transforming security forces, supporters of failed states should insist on objective international standards (e.g., civilian control, depoliticization), justifying capabilities according to explicit missions, justifying resources according to required capabilities, and providing for broad demographic representation in both officer and enlisted ranks. Standards will not only help produce better decisions about whether and how to dissolve or reform, but also will improve the prospects that the resulting forces will be effective.

Response: Abolishing Militias. Militias testify either to the state's inadequacy in providing security or its use of nonstate forces to advance special political interests. Militias may contribute to public security, but their lack of accountability and their alternative reporting chains make them, at best, obstacles to a legitimate state's control over force. At worst, they can be undisciplined, dangerous to the state, and threatening to some segments of the population.[4] Even when militias play a broadly positive role in security, it is far better to direct resources and personnel away from them and toward building adequate and accountable state forces.

The orderly demobilization of militias should be a standard policy "package" in failed-state recovery strategies, recognizing that the urgency and method of implementation will vary from case to case. The package should consist of

- clear and enforceable laws
- an agreed-upon disarmament and demobilization schedule
- reintegration and rehabilitation programs, provided for all excombatants (e.g., training and education, job placement services, recruitment into state security services).

Reintegration is essential. For militias, as for other excombatants, demobilization without reintegration risks renewing the failed-state cycle.

Response: Transforming Security Institutions. If the agencies that control security—department and ministries of defense, interior, justice, and intelligence—are not reformed, state power will remain subject to abuse, even if security forces are rebuilt and militias abolished. Often, as was the case in Iraq, Liberia, and the DRC, these power institutions are primary contributors to the insecurity and violence that lead to or exacerbate state failure in the first place. Whether they have abused or simply failed to exercise control over armed forces, such agencies often perpetuate the vicious failed-state cycle. Accordingly, they should be demolished and new ones built from scratch. This can be risky for new political leaders, especially when the old power players control the armed forces. External intervention—peacekeeping or more forcible action—may be needed to break that control.

Once the control of old power institutions is broken, intense efforts are required to design and build new institutions, staff them with able and responsible people, and write the laws and

---

[4] In post-Saddam Iraq, for example, Kurdish militia fighters (or *peshmerga*) provide important security functions and are effectively under the control of legitimate Kurdish regional leaders. But they are also active in harassing Arabs in the contested city of Kirkuk. Shi'ite militias include the quasiaccountable Badr Corps and the more troublesome and audacious Mahdi Army.

regulations that govern their operation and establish their control over armed services—which need to be rebuilt at the same time. Such security-sector reform has been addressed in a burgeoning literature, both official and academic. However, it has been unevenly implemented. Much greater attention has been devoted to restructuring police and military forces than to the organizations charged with managing them or to developing and implementing the decision-making statutes and mechanisms that provide for responsible political control.

Plans to demolish old security institutions and build new ones in their place must be drawn up, agreed to by the new government and its principal international backers, and executed under the closest possible attention.[5] There should be both an internal oversight body and one that also includes external actors. Such plans should set the foundation for

- new laws—constitutional, if necessary—to establish institutional responsibilities and roles
- clear chains of authority and command
- balance of power among ministries
- resource controls and accountability mechanisms
- unambiguous oversight of intelligence and cooperation between intelligence and armed services.

Response: Rebuilding Justice Systems. The justice system is just as important to security as the police and military forces. Without sound justice processes, law-breakers will be either released back onto the street or incarcerated without due process, perhaps indefinitely. The population is unlikely to cooperate with police and other security forces unless it perceives the justice system to be *both* effective and fair.

Any state's legitimacy rests heavily on its justice and correction systems. Yet ineffective and corrupt justice systems are commonplace in failed states. The former U.S. military commander in Afghanistan declared that the Afghan government was "extraordinarily weak" in the administration of justice. In his assessment, the lack of courts and correction systems, and insufficient U.S. and international support in these areas, was contributing to a "potentially irretrievable loss of government legitimacy."[6] Similar assessments could be made of Liberia, Sierra Leone, Iraq, Somalia, and most other failed states.

The development of a justice system is a daunting task, especially when none exists on which to build. It includes efficient and open courts; trustworthy judges and other court officers; sound processes for investigation, trial, and appeal; proper detention processes; adequate and decent penal facilities; security of justice personnel and facilities; and education of law enforcement officers in law, not just enforcement. Because building justice systems often greatly exceeds the capabilities of most failed states, supporting countries and organizations must be able to provide assistance in training and educating local officials, developing information systems, and ensuring the safety of judicial officials. The rebuilt system must be responsive to local history and customs. For example, the nation might require a religion-based justice system. In providing assistance, foreign governments and international organizations will need to understand local religious, political, ethnic, tribal, and other issues.

---

[5]   For a practical example, see Gompert et al. (2007).

[6]   U.S. Department of Defense, Office of the Assistant Secretary of Defense (Public Affairs), "News Briefing with Lt. Gen. Karl Eikenberry," transcript, December 8, 2005.

Removing Incentives for Violence

Critical Challenge 3: Fairly and Appropriately Distributing Assistance

Almost by definition, failed states are divided along ethnic, religious, or political lines. When the violence stops, the cleavages remain, and thus the chances are high that the state will once again fall into violence. To break the failed-state cycle, both immediate humanitarian aid and longer-term development assistance must be furnished in a way that does not provide incentives for continued violence. Meeting the challenge of fairly and appropriately distributing assistance requires a more demanding—and perhaps costlier—approach than is customary. But the usual approach—which is often the path of least resistance—also risks ultimately becoming the path to renewed insecurity and violence.

Response: Distribution of Humanitarian Aid. Virtually no failed or postconflict state is self-sufficient in terms of the provision of food, water, and other critical commodities when it begins the process of rescue and reconstruction. Providing assistance in those commodities is generally both popular and relatively cheap for donors, and a range of international donors have experience in providing such assistance. The rub is that virtually nothing about rescuing failed states can be purely humanitarian. Food and water are power. The first challenge in distributing humanitarian assistance is to ensure that it is not hijacked by an armed faction—either to be used directly as a coercive instrument or turned into money to buy weaponry.

Even when hijacking is avoided, providing security to aid deliverers can imperil the potential benefit to intended aid recipients. The easiest way to ensure the security of aid deliverers is to distribute aid—not just food, but all humanitarian assistance—from a few large depots that can be well guarded, preferably close to the air- and seaports where aid arrives, so the vulnerability of convoys can be reduced. Yet this easy solution spawns problems. It may make aid recipients vulnerable to crime as they travel to seek the aid or return home after receiving it. It also gives advantage to those who live close to aid-distribution centers over those who do not. If that favoritism coincides with existing divisions in society—for instance, if one political faction is primarily urban, another primarily rural—the bias is compounded. And it almost surely will breed refugee camps around distribution centers, perhaps providing handy targets for violence and adding to the burden of resettlement later. Over the longer term, it will undermine chances for local production and local markets, and it will create a culture of dependence.

Humanitarian aid distribution, as it usually occurs, is often both demeaning and dangerous for the citizens it aims to empower. Better policy would be, first, to provide aid where the people are. Aid should be delivered village to village, to avoid forcing people to leave their land in search of help. The use of community councils would be a practical mechanism for delivering aid locally while building local empowerment.[7] Distributing aid more evenly throughout the country, however, is not sufficient. The nature of the aid must also contribute to the potential of the people if the failed-state cycle is ultimately to be broken. To achieve this goal, one policy could be to bundle aid with tools for capacity building. For example, food aid could be bundled with seeds, fertilizer, and training.[8]

---

[7]   Sarah Cliffe, Scott Guggenheim, and Markus Kostner, *Community-Driven Reconstructions as an Instrument in War-to-Peace Transitions*, World Bank CPR Working Paper No. 7, Washington, D.C., August 2003.

[8]   Tom Epley lays out the suggestion in *The Plague of Good Intentions*, draft manuscript.

Each dollar of the aid might be divided as follows:

- $0.20 for food
- $0.15 for seeds
- $0.25 for fertilizers
- $0.15 for training
- $0.25 for logistics for local delivery.

Conceived as part of a capacity-building package, food aid would be empowering as opposed to dependence creating. Security and development could become mutually reinforcing rather than conflicting: Recipients would be more secure than if they had to travel for aid or live in refugee camps, and, in their homes, they could be on a path to self-sufficiency, not reduced to long-term dependence on handouts.

Security aside, existing relief agencies are mostly in the business of and thus organized for providing food and other aid—not developing agriculture or other means of national self-sufficiency. To be more effective, such organizations need to become less narrowly specialized or need to build closer partnerships with experienced development organizations. Many relief agencies are already reaching beyond pure humanitarian assistance and, in doing so, should strive toward increasing the population's self-sufficiency. Relief agencies are often the first on the ground; with enhanced skills and closer partnerships with development agencies, they would be in a better position to start laying the groundwork for breaking the failed-state cycle.

Response: Distributing Foreign Assistance. For longer-term development assistance and for regional economic development, the goals are similar: to do both in ways that build confidence in government and begin to empower communities and individuals. How development assistance is managed and distributed can enhance or imperil confidence in government and can enhance or undermine the effectiveness of aid. For example, if development assistance is funneled entirely through the central government, it can be fairly distributed across the country according to well-developed country plans or wasted away through internal corruption and greed.

To empower the citizens of failed states, a concerted effort must be made to rebuild local and regional institutions that have the capacity to receive aid and implement programs to support renewal at the local level. In general, care also should be taken to distribute development aid relatively equally across ethnic, religious, and other groups to help ensure that the assistance helps quell, not inflame, violence. Adjustments can be made if policies adopted for other reasons fall most heavily on particular groups—for instance, on Afghani farmers whose poppy crops were slated for eradication.

The central government will necessarily play an important role in the development planning process. Yet most of the success stories in failed states—from microcredits to advances in agricultural productivity—happen at the local level; they depend on empowering citizens to take the risks of changing practices. Thus, any development-planning process needs to build in a wide scope for local and regional initiative. Depending on the fault lines in particular regions, regional planning might become a way to overcome ethnic, religious, or other differences by focusing on common interests.

Critical Challenge 4: Building an Inclusive and Representative Political System

Viewed in the light of divided societies, the challenge of building political systems that include, rather than exclude, and that are accountable is not just a "good" or "democratic" initiative. It is critical in breaking the cycle of failure and violence that is itself a critical security threat. If citizens, especially citizens denominated in some way by group, feel excluded, they will feel disempowered and will seek power in other ways—perhaps by turning to violence.

Response: Strengthening the Accountability of the Government. Many failed states are highly centralized in their capital cities because of migration from the countryside and, sometimes, because of the simple lack of easy communication with the rest of the country. As a result, strategies—for assistance, reconstruction, and even security—often are very nation-centric and thus top-down. Yet most citizens perceive governance, or the lack thereof, most intensely in their towns and cities. Therefore, it is important that the national government is inclusive, not exclusive, but this is not enough. Strategies also need a strong bottom-up focus on developing local government and its accountability to its constituency.

There is no silver bullet for building accountable government. It requires a range of coordinated initiatives. For instance, distributing humanitarian and other aid throughout the country, not just in a few central locations, not only can increase the safety of citizens, it also requires local governments to oversee the process. Moreover, development assistance and planning with a strong local and regional component, as described in the previous challenge, will also build accountability close to home.

So, too, anticorruption efforts will have to be applied both from the top down and from the bottom up. With a new government, reforms and restructuring at the national level will naturally take temporary precedence. It is likely, for instance, that national civil-service reforms will need to be introduced, anticorruption laws developed and enacted, and inspection, accounting, and auditing functions created and implemented. As quickly as possible, however, it will be important to devolve such governance reforms down to the provincial and local levels and to provide provincial and local levels of government with appropriate resources and authorities. Such efforts should be accompanied by strong anticorruption laws, which should be enacted and enforced at all levels of the government. National and regional inspection, accounting, and auditing practices should be designed to ensure the appropriate allocation of resources and use of public funds.

Response: Encouraging Participation in Local Government. Focusing on free and fair elections at the national level is important, but this must be supplemented by means for local government participation. It is at the local level that most citizens will experience governance (or lack thereof). Moreover, in some countries, especially failing ones, effective and legitimate centralized government may be unrealistic. Neither Afghanistan nor the DRC can recover without good governance at the local, district, and provincial levels.

Aside from local elections, governments should be encouraged to start holding "town meetings" to solicit local development ideas and priorities. They would have the explicit purpose of including citizens and eliciting broad ideas and, in the process, building civil society. Local, community initiatives coming out of such processes could feed into the national development planning process and at the same time build local participation and buy-in. Further, funds for local and regional development should be allocated to local and regional governments once plans for their use are submitted and approved, creating a cycle that empowers and continues to empower the country's citizens.

Allocating resources to local governments will be intensely political and controversial, reflecting ethnic and other cleavages that bedevil failed states. To the extent that local regions are more homogenous than the nation, however, local initiative and participation can be more easily encouraged. And even when localities or regions are divided, regional projects for water, sanitation, electricity, and other necessities can permit common interests to be recognized.

Establishing Security for Economic Recovery

Critical Challenge 5: Securing the Nation's Productive Assets

Securing the nation's key assets addresses the failed-state cycle on all three fronts by restricting dissident-group access to assets that can fuel violence, by improving the perception that the government can meet the needs of its people, and by facilitating economic development opportunities for the population as a whole. The ability of the government to secure the state's economic resources is an essential first step in providing economic opportunities to citizens and foreign investors. Addressing this challenge entails protecting natural resources, securing public and trade infrastructure, and providing support for state security services.

Response: Protection of Natural Resources. Control of a country's economic resources often drives political struggles.[9] Collier notes that a country's dependence on primary commodity exports is strongly linked to the risk of rebellion, because primary commodity exports are the most easily looted.[10] Examples include the trafficking of blood diamonds in the Mano River Basin in West Africa and the control of mines and rubber plantations under Charles Taylor's National Patriotic Front of Liberia.

Natural resources finance conflict by funding opposition groups that manage to gain control of them. When dissidents control natural resources, not only is their power enhanced, but that of the government is diminished. The lessening of the government's ability to meet the basic needs of its citizens can further inflame antigovernment sentiments and garner public support for dissident causes. By the same token, government revenues from these resources are also critical to financing the government's side of the conflict. For example, diamond concessions were used by Sierra Leonean presidents to pay for mercenaries to provide security. And as president of Liberia, Charles Taylor used timber concessions to ensure a steady supply of arms and financial support for his security forces.

If the failed-state cycle is to be broken, it is crucial that the government establish control over its natural resources. This requires developing government agencies and security structures that effectively manage and secure the state's resources and may require the forced removal of opposition groups, as in the case of the Liberia Forestry Development Authority, which had to clear poachers and rebel groups from government-owned forest land. In addition, it requires reviewing concessions that were made under the preceding administration for the legality and potential security threats of those arrangements.

Once government control is restored, it must be sustained through regular patrolling. In many situations, geography necessitates that national security institutions enlist help from local communities—either through local community police or other trained groups. This can

---

[9] William Reno, *Warlord Politics and African States*, Boulder, Colo.: Lynne Reinner, 1999.

[10] Paul Collier and Anke Hoeffler, *Greed and Grievance in Civil War*, World Bank Policy Research Paper No. 2355, Washington, D.C., May 2000.

be part of a virtuous cycle to the extent it builds local capacity and accountability, but it also carries the risk that local police or private security forces will instigate renewed violence and human-rights abuses—an all-too-familiar problem in failed states. Such activity can be quelled by adequate support and incentives for security services, as we address next.

Response: Security of Public and Trade Infrastructure. Conflict in failed states often destroys public infrastructure, both directly through sabotage and indirectly through neglected maintenance. For example, when Liberia emerged from civil conflict, there was no electricity (even in the capital city), there was very limited communication infrastructure, and the road network was in general disrepair.

Like natural resources, public and trade infrastructure is often targeted by instigators of violence. The use of radio transmissions to spread hate messages prior to and during the Rwandan genocide is a striking example. Inadequate or insecure infrastructure symbolizes a lack of government capacity, hinders economic activity, and can impede security. For instance, the lack of electricity, combined with a lack of basic equipment, such as flashlights, deterred Liberian police from patrolling, particularly in rough neighborhoods.

By contrast, if infrastructure, such as roads and ports, can be secured and kept in working order, goods can be traded, both at home and abroad; government services, such as health care, can be delivered; and security forces can more easily patrol the country. In addition, adequate and secure roads enable individual citizens to move freely throughout the country, improving the quality of daily life through access to employment, friends and relatives, and social services.

Secure and functioning utilities and communication infrastructure also improve quality of life, foster confidence in the government, and promote security: Twenty-four-hour electricity increases the potential hours for work and study and eases the burdens of heating and cooking. And communication can enhance agricultural productivity by allowing farmers to become better informed of market prices and to develop networks with other buyers and sellers across the country. Secure infrastructure also is critical to foreign investment, which provides both jobs to citizens and revenue (through taxation and business licenses) to the government. These positive impacts compound over time, as additional investors and businesses are encouraged by the presence of others.

Response: A Visible and Professional Police Force. Policing is an important component of law, order, justice, and security, and the police force must play a central role in protecting the nation's key assets. A trustworthy and visible police force is essential for keeping local insurgent groups in check, securing natural resources and critical infrastructure, and ensuring safe economic activity. However, residents of failed states have become accustomed to unsafe environments and often have lost trust in the police. In failed, corrupt governments, police are as likely to be working for opposition groups or for the government's special interests as they are for the people.

Ensuring civilian control and local trust of the police force are not simple goals, particularly when members of the new police force were (or still are) associated with the very groups threatening public safety. Whether the force is being reformed or built from scratch, significant resources will need to go into police training. Training should include, but go beyond, traditional police training to include community relations and community policing principles, tools, and techniques.

A separate training budget will need to be established for at least the first three post-conflict years. In addition, resources will be required for standard needs. RAND's *The Begin-*

ner's Guide to Nation-Building[11] estimates the cost per police officer, including personnel, equipment, facilities, operations, and oversight, to be approximately 3.2 times the per capita GDP. Although significant, these expenditures are necessary. Ill-equipped security forces will not meet the basic security needs of the populace but will instead bolster the confidence of dissident groups and criminals. For example, in postconflict Liberia, police officers reported not having basic communication equipment, or even flashlights, for their patrols in Monrovia, much of which lacked electricity. That led to a sharp rise in crime and activities of local vigilante groups—both of which discredited the government in the eyes of the people.

Moreover, if security forces are ill paid, they will be tempted to resort to extortion or abuse to supplement their wages, leading not only to a deterioration of the security situation but also to the loss of crucial community support. In the immediate aftermath of conflict, with financial institutions in tatters, alternative methods for salary disbursement to police and other civil servants may be necessary, such as a system of "pay masters" who deliver cash payments throughout the country. In Iraq, for example, the U.S. military was able to effectively pay Iraqi government employees this way.

A community policing approach is important to ensure in-depth local knowledge among the police force and to build a sense of renewed trust between police and local community members. Adequate policing in each community calls for quantity, but quality should not and cannot be compromised. New or reformed police forces, organized around community policing, should stress quality, reliability, training, discipline, and leadership over sheer numbers.

Critical Challenge 6: Providing Security for Foreign Direct Investment

The long-term economic success of failed states rests on attracting investments that are beneficial not only for foreign investors but also to the government and its people. Yet failed states face a cruel paradox: While they need foreign investment the most, their inherent problems—poorly educated workers, limited financial resources, lack of security, and, often, rampant corruption—dissuade foreign investment. Therefore, in rescuing failed states, more attention needs to be paid to attracting foreign investment early and to developing oversight and regulatory mechanisms to ensure benefits to the government and its citizens.

In failed states, poor governance and insecurity often lead to foreign investment deals that benefit the investors and corrupt government officials at the expense of the local populace. In countries with natural resources and existing foreign direct investment, all that may be required are initial steps to review and renegotiate existing contracts to ensure that they foster a vibrant economy, engaging already-present international actors in fiscal reform and economic reconstruction. However, more innovative and aggressive measures are required in countries with little to no foreign investment. Economic growth in postconflict nations often rebounds significantly in the first or second year after the end of a conflict—partially dictated by steep declines in output during conflict.[12] The United States Institute of Peace argues that the usual delays of several years from the end of conflict for substantial foreign investment is an enormous missed opportunity to take advantage of this "golden hour." The institute suggests a rethinking of U.S. and other foreign state policy to support and protect earlier foreign invest-

[11] James Dobbins, Seth G. Jones, Keith Crane, and Beth Cole DeGrasse, *The Beginner's Guide to Nation-Building*, Santa Monica, Calif.: RAND Corporation, MG-557-SRF, 2007.

[12] Previous RAND work has found an average growth rate of 18.3 percent in a sample of 13 postconflict nations since World War II (Dobbins et al., 2007).

ments in postconflict societies so as to maximize the potential for stability and lessen the risk of a renewed failed-state cycle.[13]

Even with such policies in place, it will be essential for the state to begin early to establish appropriate governance structures and institutions to support foreign investment and other economic activity. For example, it will be crucial for recovering states to develop and implement trade agreements; establish and enforce commercial, contract, and property laws; establish banking and credit institutions; and ensure that legitimate investments are protected from threat and interference. In addition, government policies should encourage local or diaspora entrepreneurship, as well as foreign investment, perhaps through tax breaks, paid employee traineeships, or attractive industrial sites and artisan villages with required infrastructure readily available. Further, contracts with and concessions for foreign investors could include provisions to increase the benefits to local workers—by, for instance, stipulating minimum levels of local labor or requirements for training local workers.

---

[13] Johanna Mendelson-Forman and Merriam Mashatt, *Employment Generation and Economic Development in Stabilization and Reconstruction Operations*, Stabilization and Reconstruction Series No. 6, Washington, D.C.: U.S. Institute of Peace, March 2007.

CHAPTER FOUR

Creating Conditions for Empowering the Population

Meeting critical challenges that lie at the intersection of violence, economic collapse, and unfit government is necessary but insufficient to break the failed-state cycle. In addition, "enabling" conditions—targeted at empowering the country's population—must be established to put the wheels of recovery in motion. For victims of failed states to become agents of progress, and thus for the cycle to truly be broken—and remain broken—three conditions must be met:

- Most immediately, the population's basic needs (potable water, sanitation, basic health care, and education) must be satisfied.
- Second, longer-term plans for sustainable human development must be devised and implemented over time.
- Finally, through such efforts, the capacity, competence, and trustworthiness of the country's government must be enhanced.

Meeting the population's basic needs and ensuring long-term development both depend on a capable, reliable, and supportive central government. By definition, failed states lack such governments. Thus, it is incumbent upon international donors and other external actors to build capacity, accountability, efficiency, effectiveness, and trust within the local government as part of all recovery initiatives. Failure in this area will ultimately result in a failed recovery effort. The evidence for this is vivid: Witness the failure of nation-building efforts of Haiti and Somalia.[1] Some important lessons have been learned:

- Externally funded efforts should bear the "face" of the state's government to build trust in the government among the people and to instill pride within the government itself.
- Recovery efforts should be conducted in partnership with the central, regional, and local governments, even if this is more difficult, costly, and time-consuming. This helps to ensure knowledge transfer, capacity building, and, ultimately, program sustainability.[2]

Building a capable and reliable government can be a long, slow process, but it is essential for breaking the failed-state cycle. To the extent possible, international agencies and other external actors should support the government (as opposed to leading the effort themselves) in

---

[1] Seth G. Jones, Lee H. Hillborne, C. Ross Anthony, Lois M. Davis, Federico Girosi, Cheryl Benard, Rachel M. Swanger, Anita Datar Garten, and Anga Timilsina, *Securing Health: Lessons from Nation-Building Missions*, Santa Monica, Calif.: RAND Corporation, MG-321-RC, 2006.

[2] Sarah Cliffe and Nicholas Manning, "Building State Institutions After Conflict," in Charles T. Call and Vanessa H. Wyeth, eds., *Building States to Build Peace*, Boulder, Colo.: Lynne Reinner, forthcoming.

building effective and legitimate state security structures, securing the nation's key assets, fairly distributing assistance, and creating conditions for local, sustainable empowerment. The best ways to support the government in the development of such capacity is much discussed. Promising approaches are those that acknowledge the need for gradual, step-by-step transitions from externally provided services to state-provided services, which allow both for the delivery of rapidly needed services early on to benefit the population and for the time required to build capable and accountable state institutions.[3] For example, a phased transition strategy could progress from NGO provision of aid to state contracting of service delivery with external management to state management of contracted service delivery to direct state provision of services.

Government Provision of Essential Public Services

Access to basic services empowers individuals to become agents of recovery and growth. Without the provision of basic services, other aid and economic recovery efforts may become futile. For example, without access to basic public health (e.g., clean drinking water, immunizations), a sicklier population will be less able and motivated to take advantage of newly opened marketplaces or microfinancing opportunities.

It is critical that the government itself be equipped, through revenue collection and the development of internal capacity, to provide essential public services. As too many examples have shown (e.g., Hizballah in Lebanon, Hamas in Gaza and the West Bank, Fuerzas Armadas Revolucionarias de Colombia in Colombia), opposition and insurgent groups are eager to step in and fill a void when the government is unable to provide its citizens with essential services. When such groups provide health, education, and protection services instead of or better than the government, they gain legitimacy, respect, and authority in the eyes of the populace. If the government fails at providing basic services to its citizens, its legitimacy and its ability to break the cycle of failure are severely threatened.

Safe Drinking Water and Basic Sanitation

To meet basic needs and improve daily well-being, the best place to start is with clean drinking water. This basic health need is particularly important for women and children, who often spend large portions of their days traveling great distances to find it. With access to clean water and sanitation, not only does health improve dramatically, but children have time to attend school and women time to work outside the home.

Safe drinking water and basic sanitation not only avert numerous illnesses and deaths, but they also significantly increase the government's credibility. Moreover, the economic benefit, primarily through gains in productive working days, is large. Depending on the region of the world, economic benefits have been estimated to range from $3 to $34 for each dollar invested.[4]

---

[3] Sarah Cliffe and Charles Petrie, "Opening Space for Long-Term Development in Fragile Environments," in Silvia Hidalgo and Augusto Lopez-Claros, eds., *The Humanitarian Response Index 2007,* New York: Palgrave Macmillan, 2008, pp. 53–64.

[4] Gary Hutton and Laurence Haller, *Evaluation of the Costs and Benefits of Water and Sanitation Improvements at the Global Level,* Geneva: World Health Organization, 2004.

In postconflict societies, resources are limited, needs are enormous, and the competition for scarce resources can be fierce. However, in the case of water, the trade-offs are not as cruel as they appear. There are low-cost solutions to unsafe drinking water and a lack of basic sanitation—solutions that can be implemented before making large investments in modern water and sewage-transport and -treatment systems.

Proven household products for treating unsafe water are practical and can be made affordable for families in the developing world.[5] The government can ensure access to these products and promote their use. In areas where insufficient water is available, national plans can be developed to truck in water. For basic sanitation, the simplest system is a network of pit latrines, which can be built at a very low cost by local community members, once they have been trained—another way to build local initiative and empowerment.

Political and programmatic support for safe drinking water and basic sanitation should come from the national government, but solutions for safe water and sanitation will be delivered and implemented at the local level. Given the breadth of the job, the government will undoubtedly require financial and technical assistance from NGOs and other international organizations, including the private sector. Ideally, NGOs or other international organizations would work in partnership with local government public health staff. Local control will help restore trust in the government and will promote local capacity for long-term recovery, program expansion, and sustainability.

Accessible Public Health and Health Care Services

A healthy society will be a safer and more productive one. In turn, improved security and economic growth will lead to better health. This important positive cycle should begin early, with the development of a basic health care delivery infrastructure. Investment in a comprehensive public health infrastructure, affording access to clinics that provide basic health services, is essential for preventing the spread of infectious disease and treating acute and chronic conditions. The challenge, however, lies not simply in building physical infrastructure, but also in developing and implementing processes for tracking and monitoring immunizations and disease outbreaks nationwide and ensuring adequate availability of public health and health care professionals to carry out the work.

Failed states often present particularly challenging conditions for rebuilding adequate public health care. For example, refugee camps with high population densities, inadequate food and shelter, unsafe water, and poor sanitation breed communicable diseases, either alone or in combination with malnutrition. Access to health care is almost always diminished in areas of particularly acute conflict, and lack of security in general often translates to shortages of essential staff (who have fled the country or are afraid to travel to work), as well as medications and equipment (due to unsafe transport routes and cutoffs from international trade). Moreover, significant portions of the population are likely to suffer mental health consequences from conflict-related trauma, and failure to address such disorders (e.g., depression, anxiety, posttraumatic stress disorder) is likely to impede the well-being and productivity of the popula-

---

[5] Two proven, cost-effective, household-level technologies to disinfect drinking water are WaterGuard, a diluted bleach product developed by the Centers for Disease Control and Prevention (CDC) and the Pan American Health Organization, and PUR®, a powdered water-treatment product developed by Procter and Gamble and the CDC.

tion over the long term.[6] Finally, many failed states have lost the majority of their professional health care workforce to migration, leaving any remaining infrastructure for health care all but useless.

The primary goal is to develop a basic public health system that provides equitable access to prevention and treatment regimens. The word *basic* is key here. Interventions must be feasible. Developing specialty mental health services to address mental health needs, for example, is unrealistic, but incorporating mental health care into primary care services should be possible.[7] The word *equitable* also is key. Like the delivery of assistance, the nation's public health and health care–delivery infrastructure must be developed equitably—across geographic regions, socioeconomic classes, tribes, and political groups—so that all citizens feel that their health and livelihood are valued as a contribution to rebuilding the country and to avoid fueling long-standing divisions and conflict.

At first, the failed state will likely need to rely on staff from the World Health Organization and NGOs to provide needed health care services, but ministry of health officials should work with them to build appropriate training, recruitment, and capacity-building programs over time. Offering training programs (locally or through exchange programs) in epidemiology, nursing, medicine, dentistry, midwifery, community health, social work, and psychology will provide education and job opportunities to many victims of state failure, as well as the essential health workforce that is needed to keep the country healthy and thriving into the future. Additionally, as the country begins to pull itself out of conflict and signs of recovery emerge, health care professionals who had fled earlier may begin to return. As in other areas, programs can encourage their return through choices in job location and discounts on health care education and training programs for their family members.

Accessible Primary Education

Like health, basic education is fundamental in providing hope for a brighter future. In countries coming out of years of conflict, many children have been deprived of any schooling. When schools are not shut down altogether, travel to school is often unsafe. Families suffering extreme poverty cannot afford school tuition, uniform, and textbook fees. In other cases, when older family members have died from conflict or disease, children are often left to fend for themselves and must choose paid work (fighting or otherwise) over education.

A government commitment to making primary education accessible and affordable to all will send a message to the people that basic education is a fundamental human right, that children must be given tools today to be agents of recovery and growth tomorrow, and that planning for recovery is a long-term commitment of the country's leadership. Government commitment, however, is only the first and simplest step. Designing and implementing universal primary education is an arduous and resource-intensive task in the postconflict setting. Schools need to be built or renovated, teachers trained and hired, salaries secured, books and

---

[6] Florence Baingana, "Mental Health and Conflict," *Social Development Notes: Conflict and Reconstruction*, No. 13, Washington, D.C.: World Bank, October 2003.

[7] RAND and the International Society for Traumatic Stress Studies have developed mental health training guidelines for primary health care providers in conflict-affected countries. See David Eisenman, Stevan Weine, Bonnie Green, Joop de Jong, Nadine Rayburn, Peter Ventevogel, Allen Keller, and Ferid Agani, "The ISTSS/RAND Guidelines on Mental Health Training of Primary Healthcare Providers for Trauma-Exposed Populations in Conflict-Affected countries," *Journal of Traumatic Stress*, Vol. 19, No. 1, February 2006, pp. 5–17.

uniforms paid for, and special programs (e.g., meal programs to keep orphaned and extremely poor children enrolled in school) developed and implemented.

As in the health care sector, the government is likely to have to rely on NGOs and other international organizations to supplement locally available financial and human resources to deliver on universal primary education. However, to the extent possible, program planning and coordination should rest in the hands of the government. In addition, schools should be built or restored throughout the country equitably—that is, based on population density and a minimum requirement for an acceptable distance between home and school.

Sustained Human Development

To improve human industry over the long term, the more immediate need to provide essential public services must be coupled with longer-term plans for sustained human development. Such development is supported by appropriate training and education and the promotion of economic growth through ensuring accessible and safe marketplaces, facilitating and controlling trade, and other economic development efforts.

Secondary and Postsecondary Schools and Training Centers

Failed states suffer an enormous gap between long-term economic needs and available skills. Skilled people may have been killed. Others will have fled the country. Still others who, under normal circumstances, would have pursued their educations and entered the workforce, will have instead spent years fighting or hiding. To build hope for the future and to assist in keeping the cycle of violence broken, investments and opportunities must be made in the training and education of the working-age and near–working-age population. This includes ensuring that schools, vocational training centers, and business centers are established or reestablished, that they are secure and safe, and that they offer useful programs that are tied to ongoing economic development and employment opportunities.

This means rebuilding not only primary education but also other existing educational institutions in the country—colleges, universities, and vocational training centers. Vocational training will be especially important initially, and those government institutions responsible for education should coordinate with those responsible for economic development to design appropriate and relevant vocational programs. Special incentives may be required for participation among particular segments of the population—for instance, excombatants, who are especially important to reintegrate into a working, productive society.

Accessible, Safe Marketplaces

In most of the developing world, the informal business sector provides the main form of employment.[8] Once security is established in failed states, nearly all able-bodied people will begin to try to eke out a living in the informal sector. The presence of informal marketplaces is often the first sign of a return to economic life as countries or regions pull themselves out of conflict, and strong informal markets lay the groundwork for the growth of more formal economic activity. In recovering failed states, marketplaces need to be made safe and secure. In addition to providing security, the government and international civilian agencies should encourage, not

---

[8] Mendelson-Forman and Mashatt (2007).

discourage, informal marketplaces and commerce when developing and implementing new or reformed commercial rules and regulations and economic development plans.

Bosnia's Arizona Market, in the city of Brcko, is an example of how the informal sector can generate postconflict economic and social recovery. The market was formed around a NATO checkpoint and received U.S. military and NATO security support in the form of law enforcement around the market area. This provided a safe trading environment in the midst of a hotly contested, narrow corridor of land linking the east and west of the Serb Republic. In 1999, a U.S.-chaired arbitration panel declared Brcko a neutral district, beyond the rule of the Muslim-Croat Federation of Bosnia-Herzegovina and the Serb Republic. Today, Brkco is a rare Bosnian success story, where former enemies live and work side by side, and investment continues to expand.[9]

Trade Facilitation and Control

The unrest and poor governance that are typical of a failed state often result in decreased trade and even trade embargoes. For example, postconflict Liberia faced restricted trade opportunities through embargoes on timber and diamonds. Potential foreign-trade partners are also often deterred from engaging in trade with recovering failed states, given their instability and relatively high risk. Trade embargoes and reluctance among trading partners present major barriers to the economic recovery of failed states. At the same time, ongoing, viable trade in failed states that funds corrupt government officials and opposition groups (e.g., blood diamond trafficking), fueling conflict, must be brought under control.

During the recovery effort, facilitating legitimate trade—either with neighboring countries or faraway lands—will bring opportunities to the country's people that may otherwise be stymied. It will ensure that critical drugs, medical equipment, and other supplies can be imported into the country; that entrepreneurs, co-ops, and business owners can sell their wares at fair international market prices; and that trade revenue is available for the betterment of the general population, rather than the privileged few or particular segments of the population.

Facilitating legitimate trade and controlling illegal trade will require near-term action on the part of the government to set up and enforce laws, policies, and structures to ensure that trade proceeds do not fall into the wrong hands but, rather, are directed toward the public good. Over the longer term, the government should pursue trade agreements aggressively and make investments to ensure adequate transportation, customs, and port infrastructure that will support trade growth into the future.

Other Economic Development Efforts

It seems only logical that improving the lives of those who have suffered from years of conflict would include programs and plans to generate economic well-being in the immediate postconflict period. Yet such initiatives are often a secondary objective in postconflict transformation agendas. Even in Iraq, despite a massive infusion of U.S. assistance, restoring livelihoods and getting people back to work remains an unresolved challenge after more than four years of occupation. Of the nearly $20 billion of U.S.-appropriated reconstructions funds, only $805 million has been used to jump-start the private sector.[10] When security issues are

---

[9]   Reuters, "Brcko—A Rare Bosnian Success Story," Aljazeera.net, November 17, 2005.

[10]   Mendelson-Forman and Mashatt (2007).

pressing, it becomes difficult to focus attention on economic development and employment prospects—but without doing so, important opportunities for breaking the cycle of violence and despair are lost.

To maintain security, employing former combatants is an early priority. Immediately postconflict, jobs can be created through necessary rebuilding (e.g., restoration of utilities, agriculture, water, roads, bridges, jails, schools, and health care facilities) and reforming (e.g., state security structures) initiatives. To the extent possible, such restoration programs should be community based, allowing residents to participate in the rebuilding of their own communities.

The U.S. and other foreign militaries can provide important on-the-ground support for quick-impact, immediate job creation to help neutralize the security situation. However, these programs are not solutions to long-term economic development and employment needs. To be effective, they must be handed off to the newly formed government, international civilian agencies, and the private sector and integrated into longer-term plans for economic development. Strategic economic growth plans should be developed at the national and local government levels to ensure widely shared benefits of growth and to link short-term job opportunities to longer-term economic development plans. Programs could, for instance, be developed to incorporate training into industry revitalization projects so that those working on rebuilding could later be employed as skilled workers in the industries that they helped revitalize.

CHAPTER FIVE

Conclusion: Institutions and Leadership

Failed states are more likely to recover if the help they receive from the international community is targeted at the cycle of violence, economic breakdown, and unfit government. Yet the international community is poorly organized to treat the very problems at the intersections of security, economics, and politics that cause this cycle. The critical challenges identified in this paper tend to fall into the gaps between security and development organizations.

Security and development organizations have different agendas, cultures, and lines of accountability. Multinational and national agencies answer to different political authorities. Out of concern for their independence, the former are often reluctant to appear to get too close to the latter. Security organizations lack experience and expertise in development, and the military is often resistant to sharing sensitive information with civilian actors. There is also a trace of condescension among soldiers for civilians who will not take orders to operate in harm's way. For their part, development organizations are largely restricted from assisting in the strengthening of security, and many of their professionals have regarded such assistance as anathema. In addition, many NGOs are reluctant or refuse to work with the military out of fear of losing perceived independence.

To some extent, the United Nations and its family of agencies stretch across security and development, but they lack sufficient resources and authority to meet the critical challenges described here. NATO has substantial capabilities in military matters, and the European Union can call upon considerable development competence and capacity; but as of 2008, the two do not cooperate at all. Moreover, institutional disconnects are found not only among multilateral institutions and between them and their national counterparts, but also at the national level: Witness the difficulties that the United States, United Kingdom, and other governments are having integrating the strategies and actions of their own security and economic agencies.[1] From Sierra Leone and Liberia to Iraq and Afghanistan, the idea that a lead country will have no cross-institutional difficulties in treating failed states has been disproved. The security-development gap is universal.

As a starting point, there is a compelling case for easing restrictions on the involvement of development organizations in security, and some efforts are under way on this front.[2] This does not mean that development organizations should provide direct financial or technical support

---

[1] In the United States, this problem has become glaring in Iraq and Afghanistan and has led to calls for major organizational reform (e.g., the Project on National Security Reform just mandated by Congress).

[2] For example, in February 2007, the World Bank instituted a new policy on rapid response to crises and emergencies, allowing its staff to participate in integrated programs for security-sector reform within areas of bank competence (World Bank, "Operational Response to Crises and Emergencies," Operational Policy 8.00, March 2007).

for security forces, which they are, in any case, not qualified to do. But they should be encouraged, indeed required, to work directly with organizations that do provide such assistance and to take security needs into account when providing general advice, budget guidance, financial support, and program plans. This would require greater understanding and competence in security matters than development organizations currently have. But it could also present development agencies with opportunities that do not exist today, e.g., increased access to and the ability to operate in otherwise unsecured environments.

Such collaboration would also present new opportunities for security institutions: clearly, development—providing nutrition, clean water, health care, mass education—can enhance stability.[3] But until security organizations heed the unprecedented call of U.S. Secretary of Defense Robert Gates to shift resources between "hard" (military) and "soft" (development) power, targeting the failed-state nexus of violence and economic collapse will be hampered by rigid budgetary boundaries.[4] Such critical initiatives as job training and placement for excombatants will remain underfunded.

Overcoming institutional gaps, barriers, and tensions is largely beyond the reach of the professionals who toil in multilateral and national agencies. Nor can any one country, including the United States, engineer an integrated, universal approach. Reducing the problem of failed states will require agreement to do so among the world's leading (donor) states: the North Atlantic and East Asian democracies and emerging economic powerhouses, such as China and India. Although these states are increasingly aware of the seriousness of the dangers posed by failed states, other threats can seem more urgent on a day-to-day basis. It will take the commitment of political leaders, motivated by a sense of global order and human responsibility, to raise the problem to a higher position on national and international agendas.

To help address the need for unified strategies and high-level attention, we recommend that the failed-state problem, as well as the most severe cases, be placed and kept for as long as necessary on agenda of the Group of Eight (G8), plus China (at least). This "G9" should, of course, work with major international institutions, especially the World Bank, the UN, the EU, and NATO. In addition to locking in commitments of the leading states to confront this problem, a G9 mechanism could oversee efforts to close the gap between security and development, both internationally and among agencies at home.

Meanwhile, more integrated analysis of the failed-state problem is needed. This paper is hardly the last word, and we hope that it inspires more work to bridge the gap between security and development, more closely reflecting the complex reality of the failed-state problem.

---

[3]   Jones et al. (2006).

[4]   Robert M. Gates, U.S. Secretary of Defense, speech at Kansas State University, Manhattan, Kan., November 26, 2007.

Countries in Alert Zone

Table A.1
Countries in the Alert Zone of the 2007 Failed States Index

Country	Failed States Index, 2007 Rank[a]	Per Capita GDP (PPP) ($) (2006)[b]	ODA ($ millions)[c] 2000	ODA ($ millions)[c] 2006
Afghanistan	8	1,348	135.97	2,999.76
Bangladesh	16	2,130	1,167.76	1,222.72
Burundi	19	677	92.6	414.92
Central African Republic	10	1,210	75.28	133.87
Chad	5	1,749	130.16	283.7
Congo, Democratic Republic of the	7	842	177.12	2,055.72
Congo, Republic of the	26	1,442	33.18	254.41
Côte d'Ivoire	6	1,680	350.75	250.98
Ethiopia	18	1,123	686.14	1,946.83
Guinea	9	2,411	152.85	163.5
Haiti	11	1,840	208.24	581.42
Iraq	2	NA	99.55	8,661.28
Kenya	31	1,357	509.94	943.4
Lebanon	28	5,775	199.26	707.29
Liberia	27	17	67.42	268.66
Malawi	29	707	446.18	668.51
Myanmar/Burma	14	2,293	105.64	146.6
Nepal	21	1,947	387.26	514.29
Niger	32	963	208.45	401.25
Nigeria	17	1,227	173.7	11,433.92
North Korea	13	NA	0	0
Pakistan	12	2,744	692.43	2,147.17

Table A.1—Continued

Country	Failed States Index, 2007 Rank[a]	Per Capita GDP (PPP) ($) (2006)[b]	ODA ($ millions)[c]	
			2000	2006
Sierra Leone	23	893	180.63	363.85
Solomon Islands	30	2,107	68.25	204.51
Somalia	3	NA	101.01	391.88
Sri Lanka	25	5,387	275.74	795.89
Sudan	1	2,781	220.39	2,058.26
Timor-Leste	20	1,670	231.27	209.73
Uganda	15	1,643	817.09	1,550.58
Uzbekistan	22	2,304	185.75	148.61
Yemen	24	1,015	262.76	284.36
Zimbabwe	4	2,488	175.83	279.84

[a] Failed States Index ratings from Fund for Peace (2007b).

[b] Per capita GDP purchasing-power parity (PPP) in 2006 U.S. dollars from IMF, World Economic Outlook Database, October 2007.

[c] ODA amounts in then-year U.S. dollars from Organization for Economic Co-Operation and Development, OECD.Stat database, Aggregate Aid Statistics, 2a. Official Development Assistance by Recipient by Country, undated.

References

Baingana, Florence, "Mental Health and Conflict," *Social Development Notes: Conflict and Reconstruction*, No. 13, Washington, D.C.: World Bank, October 2003. As of March 4, 2008:
http://siteresources.worldbank.org/DISABILITY/Resources/280658-1172610662358/
MentalHealthConfBaingana.pdf

Cliffe, Sarah, Scott Guggenheim, and Markus Kostner, *Community-Driven Reconstruction as an Instrument in War-to-Peace Transitions*, World Bank CPR Working Paper No. 7, Washington, D.C., August 2003. As of March 4, 2008:
http://lnweb18.worldbank.org/ESSD/sdvext.nsf/67ByDocName/Community-drivenReconstructionasanInstru
mentinWar-to-PeaceTransitions/$FILE/WP+No+7+aug21.pdf

Cliffe, Sarah, and Nicholas Manning, "Building State Institutions After Conflict," in Charles T. Call and Vanessa H. Wyeth, eds., *Building States to Build Peace*, Boulder, Colo.: Lynne Reinner, forthcoming.

Cliffe, Sarah, and Charles Petrie, "Opening Space for Long-Term Development in Fragile Environments," in Silvia Hidalgo and Augusto Lopez-Claros, eds., *The Humanitarian Response Index 2007*, New York: Palgrave Macmillan, 2008, pp. 53–64.

Collier, Paul, V. L. Elliott, Håvard Hegre, Anke Hoeffler, Marta Reynal-Querol, and Nicholas Sambanis, *Breaking the Conflict Trap: Civil War and Development Policy*, Washington D.C.: World Bank and Oxford University Press, 2003. As of March 4, 2008:
http://go.worldbank.org/6BH1RL0GH0

Collier, Paul, and Anke Hoeffler, *Greed and Grievance in Civil War*, World Bank Policy Research Paper No. 2355, Washington, D.C.: World Bank, May 2000. As of March 4, 2008:
http://go.worldbank.org/V1SX8OJLX0

Dobbins, James, Seth G. Jones, Keith Crane, and Beth Cole DeGrasse, *The Beginner's Guide to Nation-Building*, Santa Monica, Calif.: RAND Corporation, MG-557-SRF, 2007. As of March 4, 2008:
http://www.rand.org/pubs/monographs/MG557/

Eisenman, David, Stevan Weine, Bonnie Green, Joop de Jong, Nadine Rayburn, Peter Ventevogel, Allen Keller, and Ferid Agani, "The ISTSS/RAND Guidelines on Mental Health Training of Primary Healthcare Providers for Trauma-Exposed Populations in Conflict-Affected Countries," *Journal of Traumatic Stress*, Vol. 19, No. 1, February 2006, pp. 5–17.

Epley, Tom, *The Plague of Good Intentions*, draft manuscript.

Fund for Peace, "Failed States Index FAQ," Web page, 2007a. As of March 4, 2008:
http://www.fundforpeace.org/web/index.php?option=com_content&task=view&id=102&Itemid=327

———, "Failed States Index Scores 2007," Web page, 2007b. As of March 4, 2008:
http://www.fundforpeace.org/web/index.php?option=com_content&task=view&id=229&Itemid=366

Fund for Peace and *Foreign Policy*, "The Failed States Index 2007," *Foreign Policy*, Vol. 161, July–August 2007, pp. 54–63. As of March 4, 2008:
http://www.foreignpolicy.com/story/cms.php?story_id=3865

Gates, Robert M., U.S. Secretary of Defense, speech at Kansas State University, Manhattan, Kan., November 26, 2007. As of March 4, 2008:
http://www.defenselink.mil/speeches/speech.aspx?speechid=1199

Gompert, David C., Olga Oliker, Brooke K. Stearns, Keith Crane, and K. Jack Riley, *Making Liberia Safe: Transformation of the National Security Sector*, Santa Monica, Calif.: RAND Corporation, MG-529-OSD, 2007. As of March 4, 2008:
http://www.rand.org/pubs/monographs/MG529/

Hutton, Gary, and Laurence Haller, *Evaluation of the Costs and Benefits of Water and Sanitation Improvements at the Global Level*, Geneva: World Health Organization, 2004. As of March 4, 2008:
http://www.who.int/water_sanitation_health/wsh0404/en/

IMF—*see* International Monetary Fund.

International Monetary Fund, World Economic Outlook Database, October 2007. As of March 4, 2008:
http://www.imf.org/external/pubs/ft/weo/2007/02/weodata/index.aspx

Jones, Seth G., Lee H. Hillborne, C. Ross Anthony, Lois M. Davis, Federico Girosi, Cheryl Benard, Rachel M. Swanger, Anita Datar Garten, and Anga Timilsina, *Securing Health: Lessons from Nation-Building Missions*, Santa Monica, Calif.: RAND Corporation, MG-321-RC, 2006. As of March 4, 2008:
http://www.rand.org/pubs/monographs/MG321/

Mendelson-Forman, Johanna, and Merriam Mashatt, *Employment Generation and Economic Development in Stabilization and Reconstruction Operations*, Stabilization and Reconstruction Series No. 6, Washington, D.C.: U.S. Institute of Peace, March 2007. As of March 4, 2008:
http://www.usip.org/pubs/specialreports/srs/srs6.html

Oliker, Olga, Keith Crane, Audra K. Grant, Terrence K. Kelly, Andrew Rathmell, and David Brannan, *U.S. Policy Options for Iraq: A Reassessment*, Santa Monica, Calif.: RAND Corporation, MG-613-AF, 2007. As of March 4, 2008:
http://www.rand.org/pubs/monographs/MG613/

Organization for Economic Co-Operation and Development, OECD.Stat database, Aggregate Aid Statistics, 2a. Official Development Assistance by Recipient by Country, undated. As of March 4, 2008:
http://www.oecd.org/document/0/0,2340,en_2649_34447_37679488_1_1_1_1,00.html

Reno, William, *Warlord Politics and African States*, Boulder, Colo.: Lynne Reinner, 1999.

Reuters, "Brcko—A Rare Bosnian Success Story," Aljazeera.net, November 17, 2005. As of March 4, 2008:
http://english.aljazeera.net/English/Archive/Archive?ArchiveID=16328

Sen, Amartya, *Development as Freedom*, New York: Anchor Books, 1999.

U.S. Department of Defense, Office of the Assistant Secretary of Defense (Public Affairs), "News Briefing with Lt. Gen. Karl Eikenberry," transcript, December 8, 2005. As of March 4, 2008:
http://www.defenselink.mil/transcripts/transcript.aspx?transcriptid=1370

World Bank, "Operational Response to Crises and Emergencies," Operational Policy 8.00, March 2007. As of March 4, 2008:
http://wbln0018.worldbank.org/institutional/manuals/opmanual.nsf/3e68bf24c2e325a18525705c001a33f2/404b870c4053068085257292001936cf?OpenDocument